www.ingramcontent.com/pod-product-compliance
Lightning Source LLC
Chambersburg PA
CBHW070426190526
45169CB00003B/1436
* 9 7 8 1 5 3 4 6 5 6 4 3 7 *